The
Kelee® Meditation
Medical Study

Troubleshooting the Mind through Kelee Meditation:
A Distinctive and Effective Therapeutic Intervention
for Stress, Anxiety, and Depression

Daniel Lee, MD

Ron W. Rathbun, Founder

THE KELEE® MEDITATION MEDICAL STUDY
Troubleshooting the Mind through Kelee Meditation:
A Distinctive and Effective Therapeutic Intervention
for Stress, Anxiety, and Depression

PRINTING HISTORY
First edition / April 2013

This study is registered at Clinical Trials.gov, NCT01527955.
Funding was provided by the UCSD
Academic Senate Grant, RK084H-LEE.
Kelee drawing copyright © 2013

ISBN: 978-0-9893432-0-6

PRINTED IN THE UNITED STATES OF AMERICA

The
Kelee® Meditation
Medical Study

Troubleshooting the Mind through Kelee Meditation:
A Distinctive and Effective Therapeutic Intervention
for Stress, Anxiety, and Depression

Daniel Lee, MD[1], Ron W. Rathbun, Founder[2]

[1]Department of Medicine, University of California, San Diego, CA
[2]Ron W. Rathbun is the Founder of Kelee® meditation and the Basic Principles of the Kelee. His theoretical research preceded this study and was used as a foundation for the set-up of this medical study. He was not involved in any aspect of this study except for the use of his theoretical work of the Kelee, Kelee meditation, and the Basic Principles of the Kelee. He did not at any time lead any of the classes, talk to the study participants, and he was not involved in the data analysis and reporting. He did do a final reading of his theory outlined in this paper for accuracy.

ABSTRACT

Context: The Kelee and Kelee meditation (KM) were developed and founded by Ron W. Rathbun. KM has not been formally evaluated for alleviating stress, anxiety, depression.

Objective: To determine effectiveness of KM on stress, anxiety, depression.

Design: 12-week, prospective, nonrandomized, mixed-methods intervention.

Setting: KM classes were held at an urban non-profit organization.

Patients: Ninety-two patients, age 18-65 years, met inclusion criteria and consented to participate, 47/92 (51.1%) completed the study.

Intervention: Participants practiced KM twice per day for 10 minutes, kept a self-reflective meditation journal, and attended 12 weekly KM classes in which participants learned about the basic principles of the Kelee and how to troubleshoot their own mind.

Main Outcome Measures: Changes in stress, anxiety, and depression were assessed through questionnaires and semi-structured interviews completed at weeks 0, 6, 12.

Primary endpoint: *a priori* change in total Depression, Anxiety, and Stress Scales-42 (t-DASS-42).

Secondary endpoints: *a priori* change in depression, anxiety, and stress subscales of DASS-42 (d-DASS-42, a-DASS-42, s-DASS-42), Beck Depression Inventory-II (BDI-II), Beck Anxiety Inventory (BAI), Perceived Stress Scale–10 (PSS-10), Symptom Checklist-90-Revised (SCL-90-R) and Short Form-36 Health Survey (SF-36).

Results: After 12 weeks, KM produced statistically significant improvements in t-DASS-42 (mean change ± standard error of the mean = 15.7±2.8, P<0.001), d-DASS-42 (4.7±1.3, P<0.001), a-DASS-42 (4.6±0.8, P<0.001), s-DASS-42 (6.4±1.2, P<0.001), BDI-II (10.0±1.3, P<0.001), BAI (5.1±1.0, P<0.001), PSS-10 (6.0±1.0, P<0.001).

Results: (*cont.*) Individual DASS subscales highly correlated with BDI-II ($\rho=0.69$, P<0.001), BAI ($\rho=0.72$, P<0.001), and PSS-10 ($\rho=0.59$, P<0.001). Global Severity Index from SCL-90-R (8.1 ± 1.1, P<0.001) and Mental Component Summary from SF-36 (10.0 ± 1.7, P<0.001) improved with KM.

Conclusions: This is the first groundbreaking study on the Kelee and Kelee meditation demonstrating an alleviation of stress, anxiety, and depression leading to an improved overall sense of mental health and well-being.

INTRODUCTION

The field of psychiatry has embraced the challenging task of studying, preventing, and treating psychological disorders and related conditions,[1-3] such as stress, anxiety, and depression, for more than 200 years.[4] Through the sequential development of a broad variety of treatment options, the current state of knowledge of how to improve mental health has evolved. However, the present need for more effective therapeutics cannot be understated.

Stress, anxiety, and depression are common within the general population as statistics suggest that nearly 26.2% of American adults (age 18 and older) suffer from a diagnosable mental disorder in a given year.[5] However, the prevalence of such disorders within populations afflicted with chronic medical conditions, including diabetes mellitus,[6,7] coronary disease,[8,9] chronic pain syndromes,[10-12] cancer,[13-14] and human immunodeficiency virus infection[15] is especially striking.

Depression, for instance, is not only more common in patients living with chronic disease,[16,17] but also has been shown to adversely impact adherence,[18-20] increase hospital re-admission rates,[21,22] and lead to longer post-operative stays.[23] In addition, patients with chronic illness often present to their general medical and mental health providers with a multitude of physical complaints (e.g., headaches, stomachaches, and fatigue) which are unexplained despite undergoing an extensive medical workup.[24] Many of these symptoms are tied to negative emotion directly related to stress,[25,26] anxiety,[27] and depression.[28] These trends underscore the magnitude and importance of mental health on physical health,[18,25,29] overall well-being,[25,30,31] and health care utilization costs.[10,18,30,32-34]

The overall well-being of any individual is impacted by the presence of negative thoughts or internal chatter.[25,26,35,36] Those who experience stress, anxiety, and depression often report having recurrent negative thought patterns.[25,35,37-40] These thoughts can exist in the form of worries, regrets, concerns, or fears about experiences in the past, the present, or the future. However, negative thoughts do not serve any useful purpose as one cannot change the past, nor predict the future. Instead, these thoughts often lead to further rumination about other related negative thoughts, which may trigger and exacerbate many of the negative feelings associated with stress, anxiety, or depression. Because negative thoughts are unresolved and disharmonious, the brain searches for resolution and understanding. Unfortunately, this leads to an ongoing cycle of repetitive thinking as the individual searches the brain's memory and its database of preexisting knowledge to find resolution, but rarely does.[41]

Naturally harmonious thoughts, however, do not cause rumination nor cause negative feelings. Instead, harmonious thoughts (such as a genuine acknowledgment and appreciation for a job well done) usually go directly into memory, without the need for the individual to further evaluate and resolve the meaning behind the positive thought.[41]

The presence of recurrent negative thoughts can lead to persistent mental distraction, difficulty focusing, and insomnia.[39,40,42,43] In addition, these negative thoughts can directly affect physiology, thereby producing a variety of physical manifestations.[25,29,31,37,44-47] It is not uncommon to develop an upset stomach,[46,48] tension headache,[49] or increased blood pressure[50,51] purely from having negative thoughts about oneself or resulting from a negative experience (e.g., argument) with another person. Studies of anxiety and depression have supported an association with hypersecretion of stress-related adrenocortical hormones, such as cortisol[29,44,52-56] and epinephrine.[29,44,52-54,56]

Newer studies[57-60] show that epigenetic changes (as manifested by DNA methylation) are induced by the chronic activation of stress hormones. Rather than restoring homeostasis, this chronic activation of stress hormones leads to numerous adverse consequences, such as impaired cognitive performance,[61,62] hypertension,[56,62,63] hyperglycemia,[46,63] and lowered immunity[29,44,52,56] and inflammatory responses.[29,44,52,53,56] To address these mental and physiological downstream effects, providers have offered multiple modalities including meditation.

Kelee Meditation

The Kelee® and Kelee meditation (KM) were developed and founded by Ron W. Rathbun.[64-67] KM is a unique and distinctive form of meditation that is easy to learn and requires only about 10 minutes twice a day to perform (Figure 1).[64-67] The goal and discipline of KM is the development of one-pointed stillness of mind. To better comprehend how KM is effective in reducing stress, anxiety, and depression, one must understand the difference between concentration and meditation, and the basic principles of the Kelee (Figures 2 & 3).[64-70]

Experiencing and understanding the distinction between brain function and mind function are of vital importance in KM. Brain function is associated with the tension-based, intellectual, thinking process and the five physical senses whereas mind function is associated with the relaxation-based, experiential, mental feeling process, self-awareness, and clear perception.[41]

Medical Model of Kelee Meditation

The medical model of KM and its effect on stress, anxiety, and depression are demonstrated in Figure 4.[65,66] Reception of incoming information (in the form of any external stimulus) occurs at the surface of the mind through our conscious awareness, often associated with our five physical senses of sight, hearing, taste, smell, and touch. The understanding of incoming information can occur in two different ways. One can *think* about the information using preconceived intellectual knowledge, or one can mentally *feel* or perceive information by using one's own perception without preconception.[64,66]

Since many people in our society tend to value the thinking process more than the feeling process, most people tend to operate purely in brain function (what one thinks) and ignore the significance of mind function (how one feels). However, when it comes to quality of life and overall well-being, it is clear that how one *feels* mentally and physically is much more important than what one *thinks*.[41]

When confronted with a new unknown experience or stimuli, being in mind function allows one to be open to perceive and truly understand something the mind has not seen before. On the other hand, being in brain function limits one to conceive using preexisting knowledge to create an understanding of what one thinks and believes. However, if the preexisting knowledge that one uses to create an understanding is false, then the conclusion that is drawn about what one experiences is similarly false. This can lead to the development of misperception, which is otherwise known as a compartment in KM.[41]

Compartments are fear-based misperceptions of life (which exist as negative thoughts and/or feelings) that may be unknowingly accepted within one's mind or that are formed about oneself in response to an external stimulus.[64-67] Throughout life, one often experiences negative external stimuli that lead to the formation or installation of compartments in one's mind.[41]

These compartments exist in the form of thought-form images. When people communicate with spoken words, the message is associated with an image representing the word, known as a thought-form image. For instance, when one thinks of an apple, one thinks of what an apple looks like, rather than visualizing the letters A-P-P-L-E. In addition, there is also a feeling behind spoken words that can be mentally sensed or perceived.[64]

Thus, when compartments form in response to negative circumstances of life, these compartments exist as thought-form images with the same negative thoughts and feelings associated with the original external stimuli. Therefore, when a similar external stimulus occurs again, this existing compartment can be triggered, which can lead to negative thoughts and feelings of stress, anxiety, or depression. It is the presence of these negative recurrent thoughts that interferes with smooth, efficient cognitive functioning (memory, concentration, and focus) and also causes insomnia and fatigue.[41]

KM guides the practitioner to reduce stress, anxiety, and depression by dissolving the associated internal negative compartments within one's mind.[64,66] Performing KM leads to the calming of brain function and opening to the experience of mind function. With continued practice, persistence, and patience, the practitioner can begin to learn on his own how to examine and understand (i.e., troubleshoot) his own thoughts and feelings from a calm, clear internal space that is free from the negative chatter and preconception associated with the brain. This increases self-awareness of the presence of internalized compartments and the practitioner begins to develop clarity of perception.[41]

Clear perception allows one to begin the process of detachment from internalized compartments which occurs through the cessation of looping followed by the processing of compartments. As each negative compartment dissipates, the practitioner experiences a subtle, but cumulative, corresponding improvement in stress, anxiety, and depression. When the flow of the Kelee is allowed to be, there is balance between the thinking and the feeling process leading to overall well-being, which leads to improved self-efficacy and reinforces the repetition of KM.[41]

Present Study

The aim of the present study was to evaluate the efficacy of KM on stress, anxiety, and depression in a chronic disease model. Our *a priori* hypothesis was that participants who completed 12 weeks of KM would demonstrate improvement in their stress, anxiety, and depression compared to their baseline assessments. Here, we present the quantitative data surrounding this research.

METHODS

This was a 12-week, prospective, non-randomized, mixed-methods study evaluating the effects of a 12-week KM class in HIV-1 infected patients on stress, anxiety, and depression. The study protocol (Project #081197) was approved by University of California, San Diego Human Research Protections Program Institutional Review Board. Research subjects provided written informed consent before participating in research activity. All clinical investigation has been conducted according to the principles expressed in the Declaration of Helsinki.

Subjects were recruited through primary care provider referrals or via flyers posted at community-based organizations. All documented HIV-infected adults of ages 18-65 years old, regardless of gender, or racial/ethnic background who expressed interest and commitment in attending a weekly KM class for the purpose of improving stress, anxiety, and/or depression for 12 weeks were eligible for participation.

Non-English readers or speakers, hearing-impaired patients, and those with literacy levels below the 5th grade reading and comprehension level were not able to participate in the study as the class, questionnaires, and interviews were only conducted in English and require reading and comprehension above a 5th grade level.

Participants were also required to suspend the use of other meditation practicesor holistic modalities during the 12-week study period in order to better attribute any changes to KM.

Assessment Measures

All study participants filled out a standard demographic and medical history survey in addition to several self-administered questionnaires including the Depression Anxiety Stress Scales-42 (DASS-42),[71] Beck Depression Inventory-II (BDI-II),[72] Beck Anxiety Inventory (BAI),[73] Perceived Stress Scale-10 (PSS-10),[74] Symptom Checklist-90-R (SCL-90-R),[75] and Short Form-36 Health Survey (SF-36)[76] at weeks 0, 6, and 12.

Participants were also asked to voluntarily participate in qualitative semi-structured interviews prior to the initial class at week 0 and after weeks 6 and 12. The interviews were digitally audio-recorded and transcribed.

CD4 lymphocyte counts and HIV-1 viral loads were obtained retrospectively near week 0 and week 12 via chart review. Study subjects were also asked to record their twice daily meditation adherence via use of 2 KM calendars, which assessed adherence for the first and last 6 weeks.

Kelee Meditation Class Structure

All meditation classes were taught by a single trained, certified instructor of KM at Being Alive San Diego (an urban non-profit ogranization), using a specific 12-week curriculum that was based on a book describing KM principles, which each participant received.[69]

Each class size was limited to a maximum of 10 subjects per 12-week session. The participants were instructed on how to perform KM at the initial session. This was followed by a comprehensive review of the Kelee principles and reference points over the subsequent 12 weeks.

At the beginning of each weekly session, a group meditation was performed, which was followed by individual introspection and contemplation. Participants recorded their observations and experiences in a KM journal.

Each participant had the opportunity to share his own journal entry and to ask questions about his own observations and experiences since starting KM. Participants were encouraged to perform the meditation practice twice daily throughout the 12 weeks of the study.

Outcome Measures

The primary outcome measure of this KM study was to evaluate the quantitative mean change in the total DASS-42 (t-DASS) score from baseline to week 12. Secondary outcome measures included assessments of the mean changes from baseline to week 12 in measurements of depression, anxiety, and stress subscales of DASS-42 (d-DASS, a-DASS, and s-DASS, respectively), BDI-II, BAI, and PSS-10, SCL-90-R, and SF-36.

Correlations between the 3 individual subscales of the DASS-42 and BDI-II, BAI, and PSS-10, respectively, were also examined.

Statistical Analysis

Since KM has never been studied before in a clinical setting, certain approximations were made in regards to the power analysis. Using an *a priori* power analysis, it was estimated that 46 subjects would be needed to complete 12 weeks of KM in order to achieve 80% power to detect a difference of 5 points in the t-DASS score with a standard deviation of 12 at an $\alpha=0.05$ (two-sided).

Statistical Analysis (*cont.*)

The investigators chose a very conservative effect size of 5 points in order to demonstrate a potentially clinically relevant and noticeable difference in participants practicing KM for 12 weeks. Assuming 20% attrition rate, we initially planned on enrolling at least 58 participants.

All statistical analyses were performed using Stata software, version 8.2 (StataCorp, College Station, Texas). All questionnaires were scored according to standard protocol.[71-77] Baseline demographic data were analyzed via univariable analyses using a t test for continuous variables and χ2 test for categorical variables. Paired t tests were performed to compare baseline to week 12 measurements.

Spearman rank correlations were calculated to evaluate the relationship between d-DASS, a-DASS, and s-DASS to BDI-II, BAI, and PSS-10, respectively. All tests were 2-tailed. A P value less than 0.05 was considered statistically significant.

RESULTS

Study Participants

Of 172 subjects screened, 106 (62%) were eligible to participate (Figure 5). A total of 92/106 (87%) subjects provided informed consent and were enrolled among ten different 12-week KM sessions from September 2008 to September 2010. Forty-seven (51%) participants completed the 12-week study including all questionnaires and semi-structured interviews. The attrition rate was 49% and the reasons for non-completion were variable.

The baseline demographic data for completers and non-completers are shown in Table 1. At baseline, completers were statistically significantly more likely to be older, highly educated, have a higher income, and own a house than non-completers.

Among completers, 66%, 53%, and 38% of participants cited having stress, anxiety, and depression, respectively, as the reason for entry into the study, which was not statistically significantly different than non-completers. There were no differences seen in CD4 lymphocyte counts, HIV-1 viral loads, or antiretroviral therapy usage between completers and non-completers. Use of antidepressants, anxiolytics, or mental health services did not influence completion rates in this study.

Meditation Adherence

Forty-five of 47 (96%) study participants voluntarily submitted their meditation adherence calendar after 12 weeks of KM. The overall 12-week mean adherence (± standard deviation) to KM was 73.3% ± 23.6% (Figure 6).

Primary and Secondary Outcomes

The primary outcome measure, t-DASS, improved significantly with a mean overall change of 15.7, $P<0.001$ (Table 2). KM also led to similar highly statistically significant mean overall declines of 4.7 ($P<0.001$), 4.6 ($P<0.001$), and 6.4 ($P<0.001$) in d-DASS, a-DASS, and s-DASS, respectively. Statistically significant improvements were also seen in BDI-II (mean decrease of 10.0, $P<0.001$), BAI (mean decrease of 5.1, $P<0.001$), and PSS-10 (mean decrease of 6.0, $P<0.001$).

In addition, 12 weeks of KM led to highly statistically significant improvements in all 9 subscales and 3 global indices of distress of the SCL-90-R. Likewise, highly statistically significant improvements in T-scores were seen in the SF-36 Health Survey in all 4 mental health scales including the Mental Component Score (MCS). Three of the 4 physical health scales also showed statistically significant improvements, but the mild improvement in Physical Component Score (PCS) did not reach statistical significance.

Correlation Analysis

After 12 weeks of KM, the overall improvements in d-DASS, a-DASS, and s-DASS were highly correlated to BDI-II (ρ=0.69, P<0.001), BAI (ρ=0.72, P<0.001), and PSS-10 (ρ=0.59, P<0.001), respectively (Figure 7).

Post-hoc Power Analysis

A post-hoc power analysis of the primary outcome measure (t-DASS) was performed with a sample size (N) = 47, significance criterion (α) of 0.05, t-DASS mean at Week 0 = 36.8 ± standard deviation (SD) of 24.2, and t-DASS mean at Week 12 = 21.0 ± SD of 19.9 with a t-DASS mean difference of 15.7 ± SD of 19.3. The estimated power in our KM study was determined to be 0.933 or 93.3%.

A post-hoc sample size calculation using our data (revised mean difference of 15.7 and power of 93.3% with an α of 0.05) resulted in an estimated sample size of only 19 participants.

DISCUSSION

The World Health Organization has defined health as "a state of complete physical, mental and social well-being and not merely the absence of disease or infirmity".[78] However, the presence of stress, anxiety, and depression can directly and adversely impact one's health and quality of life.[17,25,29-31] Quality of life is ultimately determined by how an individual mentally *feels* about himself and the world around him. It is not determined by what an individual *thinks* about himself or by the number of material possessions that one acquires.[41]

For instance, when a person does not mentally feel well, rarely does that person feel physically well or experience a high quality of life. This occurs because mental health (a function of the mind) actually precedes physical health (a function of the brain).[64,66,68] It is often observed that young children have a sense of freedom (associated with quality of life), which comes from operating from the feeling process (mind function) rather than the thinking process (brain function).[41]

However, as children "grow up", use of the brain and intellect are emphasized and revered, which overshadows how one feels. Over time, this imbalance may lead one to feel more disconnected as daily life decisions are dictated by preconceived thoughts, ideas, and beliefs (compartments) rather than by how one truly feels.

Stress, anxiety, and depression form and a decline in quality of life ensue.[41]

On the other hand, true quality of life occurs when the mind (what one feels) precedes the brain (what one thinks), which controls the physical body (what one does). KM allows one to develop mind function to complement brain function so that what one feels and thinks are not in opposition. This is the key to improving quality of life.[41]

Science has always focused its attention on the effect of mental and physical tension in causing disease in the human body,[31,45,47,79] but rarely has science looked at the influence and power of relaxation on mental and physical health. Health care providers commonly instruct patients to relax, but how does one truly relax? The answer lies in learning how to still the mind. In KM, stillness of mind is synonymous with mental and physical relaxation, which is the opposite of tension. Tension in the physical body can manifest in many different ways, such as headaches, stomachaches, or muscle/joint aches.[31,64,66,80]

Longstanding tension in the physical body may progress to the development of chronic conditions, such as hypertension,[53,63,81] peptic ulcer disease[46,53,81,82] or arthritis.[81] KM provides a powerful technique for each individual to begin to disengage from the mental tension associated with brain chatter and experience true mental relaxation through one-pointed stillness, which begins to reverse the deleterious effects of mental and physical tension on the body and improves overall quality of life.[41]

KM offers a new scientific paradigm in the understanding of stress, anxiety, and depression. Each person's mind experiences external stimuli from interaction in the outside world, as well as internal stimuli from one's own thoughts. Anything that is not understood or misunderstood in the mind (resulting from both external and internal stimuli) becomes compartmentalized in a negative thought-form image, which is associated with mental tension.[64-66,68] This mental tension leads to the release of stress hormones thereby causing the typical physiological manifestations of stress.

Depending on the nature and degree of the stress, symptoms may range, for example, from a minor heart arrhythmia to mild chest pain to a severe, life-threatening myocardial infarction. As stress mounts and mental looping persists in an attempt to understand the stimuli or situation, increasing mental energy can become compressed into fear and/or worry-related compartments.[64]

Anxiety forms when a person does not know how to mentally deal with fears and worry. The mental energy within the fear or worry-related compartment cannot always be contained and spills over into the physical body. Thus, anxious persons tend to manifest with a high energy state associated with adrenaline or the "fight-or-flight" response. However, the physical body has a limited supply of energy which eventually depletes, thereby causing mental and physical fatigue.[64]   If an individual is not able to mentally deal with stress or anxiety, anger may develop.   If these anger-related compartments are directed inwards towards oneself, depression can occur.[41]

Depression forms when a person believes someone else's negative opinion of him or creates his own negative opinion about himself.[64,66,68] Over time, looping through depression-related compartments drains mental and physical energy leading to a low energy state commonly seen with depression.[64,66,68]   Ultimately, it is the presence and unique combination of these internal negative compartments that define stress, anxiety, and depression for each individual.[64,66,68]

The initial step of KM focuses on quieting the unresolved thoughts associated with internal brain chatter, which often interferes with smooth cognitive functioning of the brain.[64,66] As one begins KM by mentally relaxing through both hemispheres of the brain, one may start to mentally feel and sense areas of tension in the lesser Kelee, which are associated with the energy of negative thoughts associated with compartments.[41]

The power of a relaxed, still mind lies in its ability to calm down the tension-filled chatter of the brain. This occurs via mentally allowing calmer, relaxed energy to comb over dense areas of tension, thus leading to dissolution of the compartments.   This is analogous to an agitated person calming down after encountering people who are calm and relaxed. Initial benefits of calming down brain function through KM include cessation of brain chatter leading to improved mental focus, concentration, memory, and sleep.[64,66]

Calming down brain function in the lesser Kelee prepares one to access mind function in the greater Kelee.[64] Stillness of mind allows one to become self-aware of one's own compartments, which leads to improved clarity and depth of perception. When trying to perceive, there exists two points of reference: a primary point (where one perceives from) and a secondary point (the object of perception). The central primary point of reference is located at a still-point within the greater Kelee and is used to perceive and understand all secondary points, including compartments.[66]

KM teaches the practitioner how to access mind function and use perception on command. Perception is a valuable tool for any person as it can be used in an inward direction to begin the process of self-understanding (or troubleshooting) one's own mind or used in an outward direction to become more aware of one's physical surroundings and understand one's interactions in the world.[41]

In the absence of using perception, one tends to ruminate endlessly in the form of brain chatter, which is otherwise known as looping. The amount of mental energy that is wasted while looping with a compartment can be enormous. In fact, looping may leave an individual with stress, anxiety, or depression feeling mentally and physically spent as energy is pulled away from the physical body to support the looping process.[64-66,68]

With KM, as clarity of perception deepens, one begins to detach from looping with compartments. As detachment starts, the person becomes less and less affected by negative thoughts and feelings associated with that compartment. Because one is not continuing to feed energy to the compartment by looping, the compartment begins to consume its own energy until it dissipates.[64-66,68]

The means by which the compartment dissipates is called processing. During processing, it is not unusual to feel some emotional discomfort or physiological effects. If a compartment was linked with emotional or physical discomfort at the time it was formed, it will mimic the same response when it processes out. However, when the compartment has dissolved, it is gone permanently and cannot be triggered again. This removal of the underlying negative trigger is what makes KM distinctive and unlike coping techniques that distract one's mental focus away from the problem or that create a new way of "thinking" about how one feels.[41]

These coping techniques may work temporarily as one consciously and purposefully uses the particular coping technique. However, once one ceases using the coping technique, one still remains at risk for re-experiencing the same negative compartment (if exposed to the same external stimulus) because the compartment still remains present and viable. KM is unique in that it removes the underlying compartments that directly cause stress, anxiety, and depression.[41]

The final step of KM involves introspection and contemplation, which allows one to learn how to troubleshoot his own mind. Introspection provides one with an opportunity to evaluate his meditation practice systematically, while contemplation allows one to open up his perception to learn and understand what is affecting his life and why.[41]

This landmark KM study has shown how a short 12-week non-pharmacologic, non-cognitive intervention used in a population with varying degrees of stress, anxiety, and depression led to highly statistical significant improvements and correlations across multiple well-established and validated instruments (Table 2, Figure 7).

The mean improvement of the primary outcome measure (t-DASS score) of 15.7 far surpassed our initial conservative estimate of the effect size of 5 points. Post-hoc analyses revealed that the actual power was quite high at 93.3% and the number or participants needed for this study was only 19 participants. Thus, future studies of KM may not need to enroll as many participants as we had anticipated (N=46) based on sample size calculations given the much larger than anticipated effect size and power of this simple intervention.

One of several notable findings was that improvements in the primary outcome measure were seen in 38/47 (81%) participants (data not shown), many of whom were also receiving antidepressant and/or anti-anxiety medications as well as receiving care from a mental health professional. This suggests that KM has clinical utility as a single modality or concurrently with other established therapies.

Although the focus of this study was on stress, anxiety, and depression, KM also produced improvements on other broader measures of mental health. Statistically significant improvements were demonstrated in a wide range of psychological problems and psychopathology including declines in overall psychological distress (measured by Global Severity Index), number of self-reported symptoms (measured by Positive Symptom Total), and intensity of symptoms (measured by Positive Symptom Distress Index) as assessed by SCL-90-R.

Furthermore, KM produced statistically significant improvements in all 4 individual measures of mental health comprising the MCS of the SF-36, which evaluated functional health and well-being from a mental and physical standpoint. Interestingly, although the PCS was not statistically significantly improved, there were several individual measures of physical health that did improve significantly, including physical functioning, role-physical, and general health. This finding is consistent with Kelee understanding that improving mental health by removing the underlying compartments (i.e., negative thoughts and/or emotions that may affect one's physiology) through practicing KM would precede and lead to the improvements seen in physical health.[64,66,68]

Potential limitations of this study include the lack of a placebo or therapeutic control arm, short study duration, single site recruitment, non-diverse study population, attrition rate of 49% (although comparable to other behavioral interventions), and potential bias due to guidance from KM teacher affecting the outcome. Future studies of KM may benefit from the inclusion of a control or placebo arm as a comparator or may involve a direct comparison study of KM with other currently well-established treatments of stress, anxiety and depression, including pharmacologic medications and psychotherapy.

Other future directions include studying KM in a variety of diverse populations, evaluating psychoneuroimmunologic effects of KM, and developing a specific KM scale or questionnaire to more accurately assess and measure changes associated with the dissolution of compartments associated with KM.

Current ongoing evaluations include examining predictors of completion status (completers vs. non-completers), predictors of clinical response to KM, 1 year longitudinal data, and review of the qualitative interviews, which will be presented and discussed in separate manuscripts in the near future.

CONCLUSION

This groundbreaking KM study was able to show how a short 5-10 minute meditation practice focused on developing stillness of mind can lead to highly statistically significant improvements in stress, anxiety, and depression in only 12 weeks. KM provides a roadmap for each individual to learn stillness, which allows one to begin to troubleshoot his own mind.

KM brings about a new paradigm shift in understanding the difference between the brain and the mind, and how each person can learn to free himself from the negative compartments that cause stress, anxiety, and depression. With continued KM practice, persistence, and patience beyond 12 weeks, the long-term potential implications of KM on truly alleviating mental health problems and its downstream effects on physical health are enormous, profound, and achievable.

Table 1. Demographic Basline Data

Characteristic	Total (n=92)	Non-Completers (n=45)	Completers (n=47)	P value[a]
Age (y), mean (SD)	46.9 (8.0)	45.2 (8.8)	48.6 (6.9)	**0.04**
Gender (%)				0.16
Male	97.8%	100.0%	95.7%	
Female	2.2%	0.0%	4.3%	
Race/Ethnicity[b] (%)				0.09
Caucasian	68.5%	60.0%	76.6%	
Non-Caucasian	31.5%	40.0%	23.4%	
Education (%)				**0.04**
<College degree	53.3%	64.4%	42.6%	
≥College degree	46.7%	35.6%	57.5%	
Marital Status (%)				0.34
Single	80.4%	84.4%	76.6%	
Married/Partner	19.6%	15.6%	23.4%	
Work Status (%)				0.16
Unemployed/Not working	66.3%	73.3%	59.6%	
Full-/part-time	33.7%	26.7%	40.4%	
Income (%)				**0.04**
<$20,000	48.9%	60.0%	38.3%	
≥$20,000	51.1%	40.0%	61.7%	
Housing (%)				**0.001**
Rent/Other	73.9%	88.9%	59.6%	
Owner	26.1%	11.1%	40.4%	
Religion (%)				
No	65.2%	64.4%	66.0%	0.88
Yes	34.8%	35.6%	34.0%	

Table 1. Demographic Baseline Data *(cont.)*

Characteristic	Total (n=92)	Non-Completers (n=45)	Completers (n=47)	P value[a]
Holistic use (%)				0.38
No	57.6%	62.2%	53.2%	
Yes	42.4%	37.8%	46.8%	
Prior KM Experience (%)				0.97
No	95.7%	95.6%	95.7%	
Yes	4.4%	4.4%	4.3%	
Other Meditation Practice (%)				0.31
No	41.3%	46.7%	36.2%	
Yes	58.7%	53.3%	63.8%	
Reason for Study Entry Depression (%)				0.15
No	54.4%	46.7%	61.7%	
Yes	45.7%	53.3%	38.3%	
Reason for Study Entry Anxiety (%)				0.99
No	46.7%	46.7%	46.8%	
Yes	53.3%	53.3%	53.2%	
Reason for Study Entry Stress (%)				0.88
No	34.8%	35.6%	34.0%	
Yes	65.2%	64.4%	66.0%	
HIV Risk Factor (%)				0.83
Gay/Bisexual (G/B)	88.0%	88.9%	87.2%	
G/B + Injection Drug Use	2.2%	2.2%	2.1%	
Heterosexual	5.4%	4.4%	6.4%	
Injection Drug Use	1.1%	2.2%	0.0%	
Unknown	3.3%	2.2%	4.3%	
HIV+ (y), mean (SD)	13.8 (8.0)	14.1 (8.1)	13.5 (8.0)	0.73

Table 1. Demographic Baseline Data *(cont.)*

Characteristic	Total (n=92)	Non-Completers (n=45)	Completers (n=47)	P value[a]
CD4 Count (cells/mm3) median (range)	491 (23-1250)	483 (23-1231)	494 (154-1250)	0.38
Viral Load (log 10 copies/mL) median (range)	1.69 (1.48-5.34)	1.70 (1.60-5.34)	1.68 (1.48-5.15)	0.34
Anti-HIV Medication Use (%)				
No	19.6%	22.2%	17.0%	0.53
Yes	80.4%	77.8%	83.0%	
Anti-Depressant Use (%)				0.22
No	57.6%	51.1%	63.8%	
Yes	42.4%	48.9%	36.2%	
Anxiolytic Use (%)				0.13
No	56.5%	64.4%	48.9%	
Yes	43.5%	35.6%	51.0%	
Mental Health Provider (%)				0.14
No	52.2%	60.0%	44.7%	
Yes	47.8%	40.0%	55.3%	
Primary Care Provider (%)				0.41
Study Investigators	27.2%	31.1%	23.4%	
Other Providers	72.8%	68.9%	76.6%	

Abbreviation: y = years, SD = standard deviation
[a]t test used for continuous variables, X2 test used for categorical variables
[b]Race/ethnicity was defined by the participant

Table 2. Effects of 12 Weeks of Kelee Meditation on Primary and Secondary Endpoints (N=47)

Outcome Measure	Baseline Score Week 0 (mean ± SEM)	Final Score Week 12 (mean ± SEM)	Overall change Week 0 to 12[a] (mean ± SEM)	P value[b]
Primary Endpoint				
Depression Anxiety Stress Scales - 42 (DASS-42)				
Total Score (t-DASS)	36.8 ± 3.5	21.0 ± 2.9	15.7 ± 2.8	**<0.001**
Secondary Endpoints				
Depression Anxiety Stress Scales - 42 (DASS-42)				
Depression Subscale (d-DASS)	12.2 ± 1.5	7.5 ± 1.3	4.7 ± 1.3	**<0.001**
Anxiety Subscale (a-DASS)	9.6 ± 1.2	4.9 ± 0.8	4.6 ± 0.8	**<0.001**
Stress Subscale (s-DASS)	15.0 ± 1.3	8.7 ± 1.2	6.4 ± 1.2	**<0.001**
Beck Depression Inventory II (BDI-II)	18.0 ± 1.5	8.0 ± 1.2	10.0 ± 1.3	**<0.001**
Beck Anxiety Inventory (BAI)	12.7 ± 1.3	7.6 ± 1.1	5.1 ± 1.0	**<0.001**
Perceived Stress Scale-10 (PSS-10)	19.8 ± 1.0	13.8 ± 1.0	6.0 ± 1.0	**<0.001**
Symptom Checklist - 90 Revised (SCL-90R)[c]				
Somatization (SOM)	61.0 ± 1.9	56.2 ± 1.7	4.7 ± 1.4	**0.001**
Obsessive-Compulsive (O-C)	67.0 ± 1.7	59.4 ± 1.7	7.6 ± 1.0	**<0.001**
Interpersonal Sensitivity (I-S)	66.4 ± 1.4	59.2 ± 1.6	7.3 ± 1.3	**<0.001**
Depression (DEP)	69.6 ± 1.2	61.7 ± 1.7	7.9 ± 1.4	**<0.001**
Anxiety (ANX)	64.8 ± 1.6	57.4 ± 1.7	7.4 ± 1.4	**<0.001**
Hostility (HOS)	56.4 ± 1.3	50.7 ± 1.4	5.7 ± 1.3	**<0.001**
Phobic Anxiety (PHOB)	59.9 ± 1.6	55.0 ± 1.5	4.9 ± 1.4	**<0.001**
Paranoid Ideation (P-I)	58.1 ± 1.8	51.8 ± 1.7	6.3 ± 1.6	**<0.001**
Psychoticism (PSY)	64.7 ± 1.6	60.0 ± 1.6	4.7 ± 1.3	**<0.001**

Table 2. Effects of 12 Weeks of Kelee Meditation on Primary and Secondary Endpoints (N=47) *(cont.)*

Outcome Measure	Baseline Score Week 0 (mean ± SEM)	Final Score Week 12 (mean ± SEM)	Overall change Week 0 to 12[a] (mean ± SEM)	P value[b]
Secondary Endpoints *(cont.)*				
Symptom Checklist - 90 Revised (SCL-90R)[c]				
Global Severity Index (GSI)	68.0 ± 1.4	59.9 ± 1.7	8.1 ± 1.1	**<0.001**
Positive Symptom Total (PST)	65.7 ± 1.3	58.9 ± 1.7	6.8 ± 0.9	**<0.001**
Positive Symptom Distress Index (PSDI)	60.9 ± 1.3	55.1 ± 1.2	5.8 ± 1.3	**<0.001**
Short Form - 36 Health Survey (SF-36)[d]				
Physical Functioning (PF)	47.8 ± 1.4	49.7 ± 1.2	1.9 ± 0.9	**0.04**
Role-Physical (RP)	40.7 ± 1.9	45.7 ± 1.8	5.0 ± 2.2	**0.03**
Bodily Pain (BP)	46.0 ± 1.7	48.3 ± 1.5	2.3 ± 1.4	0.11
General Health (GH)	42.9 ± 1.8	48.1 ± 1.7	5.2 ± 1.0	**<0.001**
Vitality (VT)	44.2 ± 1.5	50.5 ± 1.6	6.3 ±1.3	**<0.001**
Social Functioning (SF)	38.5 ± 1.7	45.2 ± 1.4	6.7 ±1.5	**<0.001**
Role-Emotional (RE)	35.2 ± 1.9	47.0 ± 1.8	11.9 ± 2.2	**<0.001**
Mental Health (MH)	41.6 ± 1.8	47.6 ± 1.7	5.9 ± 1.5	**<0.001**
Physical Component Summary (PCS)	47.4 ± 1.7	48.5 ± 1.4	1.1 ± 1.2	0.34
Mental Component Summary (MCS)	37.2 ± 1.8	47.2 ± 1.8	10.0 ± 1.7	**<0.001**

Abbreviation: SEM = standard error of the mean

[a] A positive score represents a reported improvement from baseline whereas a negative score represents a reported decline from baseline.

[b] Paired t tests were performed.

[c] All scores are reported as T-scores with a mean of 50. Lower scores indicate better health.

[d] All scores are reported as T-scores with a mean of 50. Higher scores indicate better health.

Figure 1. How to Perform Kelee Meditation

Kelee meditation is composed of 3 steps, which take a total of approximately 10 minutes to perform. Step 1 takes 2 minutes to perform and involves mentally relaxing the brain network and calming down the brain chatter associated with the lesser Kelee. Step 2 involves further mental relaxation thus allowing the conscious awareness to drop into the greater Kelee and maintaining one-pointed stillness of mind for 3 minutes. Introspection and contemplation comprise Step 3, which takes up to 5 minutes.[65,66]

Step 1
(2 minutes)

1. Close your eyes and mentally start to relax.

2. Locate and mentally feel your conscious awareness at the top of your head.

3. From the top of the head, mentally relax your conscious awareness into a flat plane of awareness. Allow this plane of awareness to soften and pass through both hemispheres of the brain, ultimately settling at the surface of the mind at eye level.

4. When the relaxed horizontal plane of conscious awareness reaches the surface of the mind, gently bring your conscious awareness to a single point of perception in the center of your head.

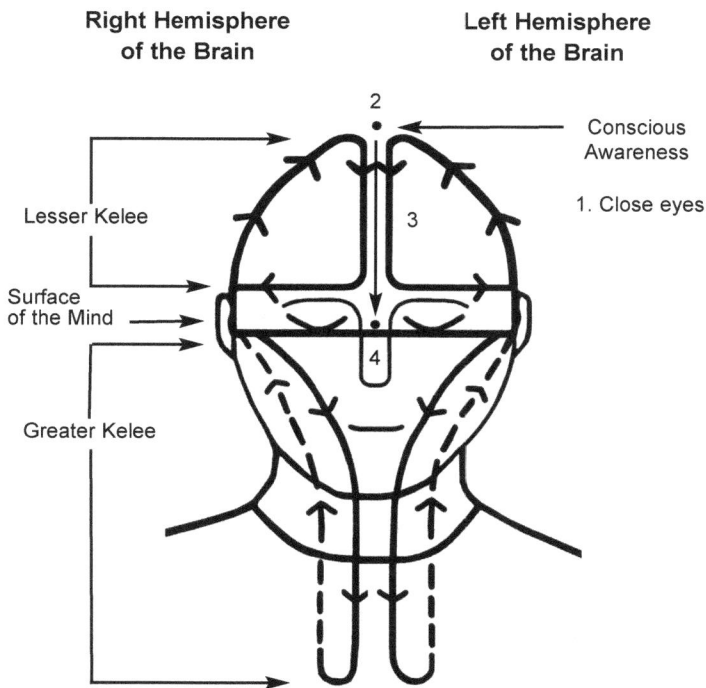

Right Hemisphere of the Brain

Left Hemisphere of the Brain

2

Conscious Awareness

1. Close eyes

Lesser Kelee

3

Surface of the Mind

4

Greater Kelee

Source: Ron W. Rathbun, *Troubleshooting the Mind: Understanding the Basic Principles of the Kelee®* (Oceanside: Quiescence Publishing, 2010) 216. Print.

49

Figure 1. How to Perform Kelee Meditation (*cont.*)

Step 2
(*3 minutes*)

5. From a single point of perception, allow your conscious awareness to drop below the surface of the mind to a natural still point within the greater Kelee.

6. Maintain stillness in the greater Kelee for 3 minutes.

7. After experiencing stillness, return to full consciousness at the surface of the mind and open your eyes.

Step 3
(*5 minutes*)

8. Upon returning from meditation, reflect on the quality of your practice through introspection and contemplation.

Source: Ron W. Rathbun, *Troubleshooting the Mind: Understanding the Basic Principles of the Kelee®* (Oceanside: Quiescence Publishing, 2010) 216. Print.

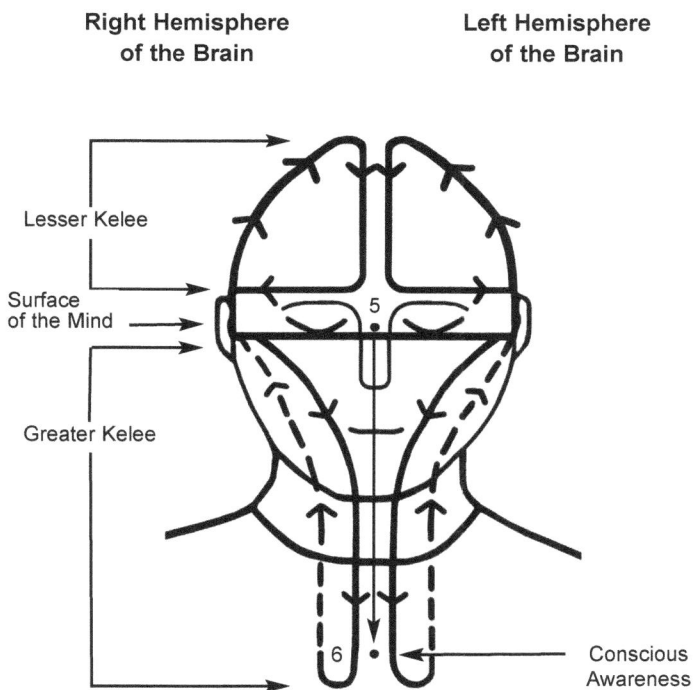

Right Hemisphere of the Brain

Left Hemisphere of the Brain

Lesser Kelee

Surface of the Mind

Greater Kelee

5

6

Conscious Awareness

Source: Ron W. Rathbun, *Troubleshooting the Mind: Understanding the Basic Principles of the Kelee®* (Oceanside: Quiescence Publishing, 2010) 216. Print.

Figure 2. Kelee Definitions

Several important key points in understanding Kelee meditation are explained, including the definition of the Kelee and the main differences between concentration and meditation.[65,66]

1. **Kelee:** Sanskrit word meaning "having to do with different states of mind; Greek and Hebrew translation means vessel or receptacle. Pronunciation "key-lee".

2. **Concentration:** Focusing without distraction, an active doing process.

3. **Kelee Meditation (KM):** A non-distracted conscious awareness (absent of thinking and the five physical senses). A mind being still of thought, an awareness of nothing, an inactive being process. Goal and discipline of KM is focused on developing one-pointed stillness of mind.

4. **Introspection:** Self-evaluation on the quality of one's meditation for retrospective and observational purposes.

5. **Contemplation:** Pondering one's observations, which provides an opportunity for self-learning.

Source: Ron W. Rathbun, *Troubleshooting the Mind: Understanding the Basic Principles of the Kelee®* (Oceanside: Quiescence Publishing, 2010) 216. Print.

Figure 3. Basic Principles of the Kelee

Understanding Kelee meditation requires knowledge of the basic principles of the Kelee, including the key reference points of the Kelee and terminology.[65,66]

1. **Conscious Awareness (CA):** Term to describe where one's conscious mental focus is directed at any moment; a point of perception between the intellectual outside physical world and the inside world of emotion.

2. **Brain Function (BF):** Thinking, analyzing, storing intellectual knowledge, and running the physical body.

3. **Mind Function (MF):** Mentally feeling as an objective observer and is synonymous with a relaxed sense of perception.

4. **Surface of the Mind (SOM):** A horizontal plane of electrochemical energy at eye level (which can be sensed with practice); a division point between the brain and deeper states of mind; a reception point for incoming information, a point of contemplation, and a place to make decisions.

5. **Lesser Kelee (LK):** An electrochemical field of energy above the surface of the mind associated with the brain, the intellect, and the thinking process.

6. **Greater Kelee (GK):** An electrochemical field of energy below the surface of the mind associated with the mental feeling process, emotion, and deeper states of mind.

7. **Compartments:** Negative thoughts/feelings (i.e., "baggage", emotional "buttons", or "issues") manifesting as nonproductive, inefficient behavioral traits.

8. **Looping:** Occurs when the conscious awareness is attached to a negative compartment, resulting in a repetitive circulation of self-destructive thoughts.

9. **Cessation of Looping:** Moving the conscious awareness out of repetitive thinking or brain "chatter" into the open clear perception of mind.

10. **Detachment:** State of being unaffected by negative thoughts and emotions.

11. **Processing:** Means by which internalized electrochemical negativity (i.e., compartments) dissipates and dissolves.

12. **Flow of the Kelee:** Occurs when the electrochemical energy of how you think and the energy of how you feel flow together in unison without beginning or end.

Source: Ron W. Rathbun, *Troubleshooting the Mind: Understanding the Basic Principles of the Kelee*® (Oceanside: Quiescence Publishing, 2010) 216. Print.

Figure 4. Medical Model of Kelee Meditation

This model shows how an external stimulus can lead to the formation of an internal negative compartment associated with depression, anxiety, and stress. Performing Kelee meditation calms brain function and opens up mind function associated with improved self-awareness and clarity of perception.[65,66]

Detachment from the negative compartment occurs through cessation of looping and processing, which then leads to the dissolution of this negative compartment and improvement in overall well-being. This leads to self-efficacy and reinforces repetition of Kelee meditation, thus leading to continued improvements in quality of life.[65,66]

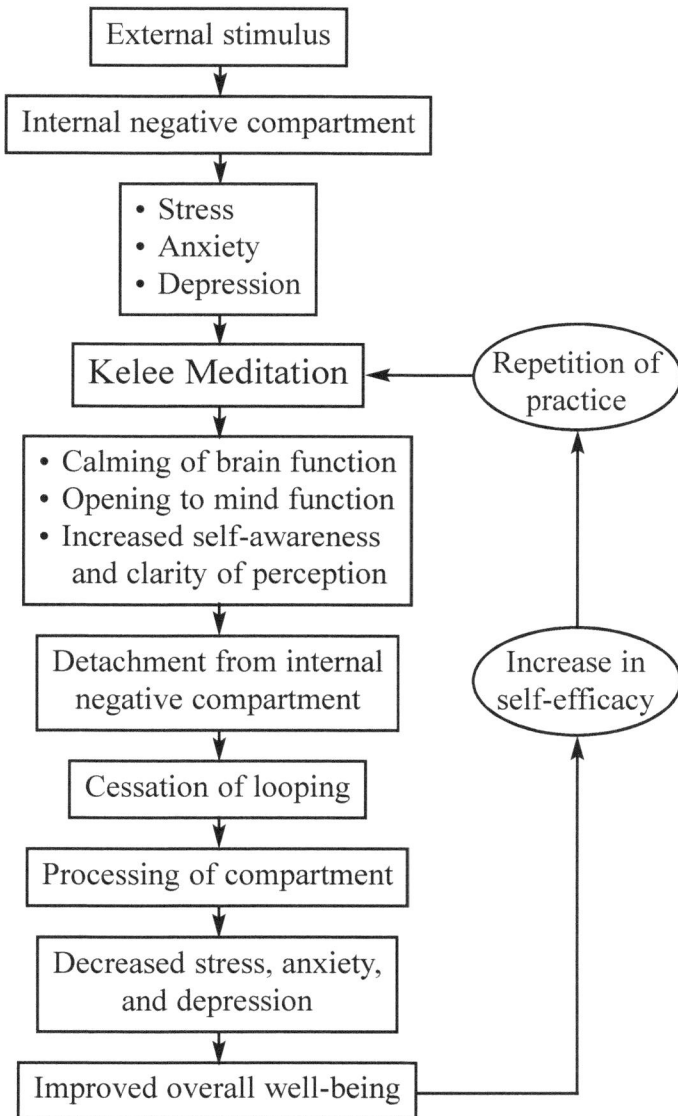

External stimulus

↓

Internal negative compartment

↓

- Stress
- Anxiety
- Depression

↓

Kelee Meditation ← Repetition of practice

↓

- Calming of brain function
- Opening to mind function
- Increased self-awareness and clarity of perception

↓

Detachment from internal negative compartment

↓

Cessation of looping

↓

Processing of compartment

↓

Decreased stress, anxiety, and depression

↓

Improved overall well-being → Increase in self-efficacy → (Repetition of practice)

Source: Ron W. Rathbun, *Troubleshooting the Mind: Understanding the Basic Principles of the Kelee®* (Oceanside: Quiescence Publishing, 2010) 219. Print.

Figure 5. Kelee Meditation Study Disposition

Disposition of subjects are shown. The screening of all 172 subjects occurred prospectively from September of 2008 to September of 2010. Reasons for ineligibility, non-consent, and non-completion are listed.

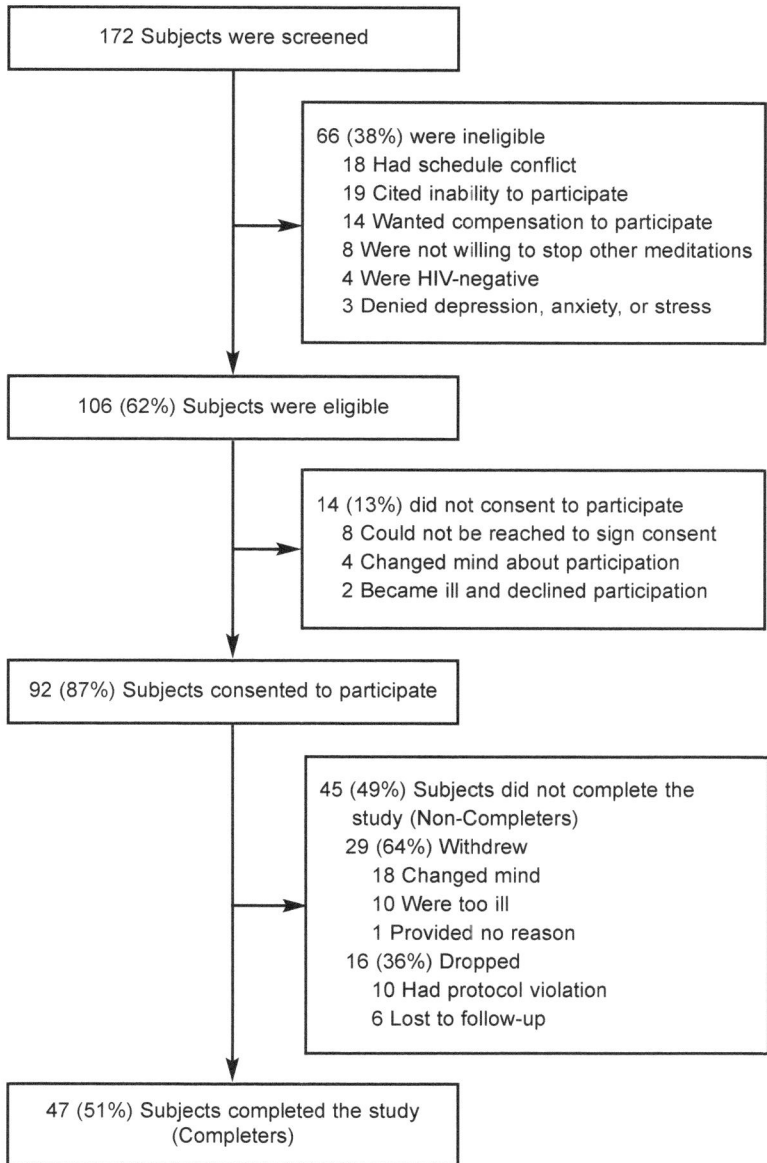

```
┌─────────────────────────────────────┐
│   172 Subjects were screened         │
└─────────────────────────────────────┘
                │
                │        ┌──────────────────────────────────────────────┐
                │        │ 66 (38%) were ineligible                     │
                │──────▶ │    18 Had schedule conflict                  │
                │        │    19 Cited inability to participate         │
                │        │    14 Wanted compensation to participate     │
                │        │    8 Were not willing to stop other          │
                │        │       meditations                            │
                │        │    4 Were HIV-negative                       │
                │        │    3 Denied depression, anxiety, or stress   │
                ▼        └──────────────────────────────────────────────┘
┌─────────────────────────────────────┐
│   106 (62%) Subjects were eligible   │
└─────────────────────────────────────┘
                │
                │        ┌──────────────────────────────────────────────┐
                │        │ 14 (13%) did not consent to participate      │
                │──────▶ │    8 Could not be reached to sign consent    │
                │        │    4 Changed mind about participation        │
                │        │    2 Became ill and declined participation   │
                ▼        └──────────────────────────────────────────────┘
┌──────────────────────────────────────────┐
│   92 (87%) Subjects consented to          │
│   participate                             │
└──────────────────────────────────────────┘
                │
                │        ┌──────────────────────────────────────────────┐
                │        │ 45 (49%) Subjects did not complete the       │
                │        │    study (Non-Completers)                    │
                │        │    29 (64%) Withdrew                          │
                │──────▶ │       18 Changed mind                        │
                │        │       10 Were too ill                        │
                │        │       1 Provided no reason                   │
                │        │    16 (36%) Dropped                          │
                │        │       10 Had protocol violation              │
                │        │       6 Lost to follow-up                    │
                ▼        └──────────────────────────────────────────────┘
┌──────────────────────────────────────────┐
│   47 (51%) Subjects completed the study   │
│   (Completers)                            │
└──────────────────────────────────────────┘
```

Figure 6. Overall Kelee Meditation Adherence During 12-Week Study Period (N=45)

Mean overall adherence (± SD) to Kelee meditation as assessed by use of self-reported calendars was 73.3% ± 23.6% in 45 of 47 subjects who completed the 12-week study. Two participants did not submit adherence data.

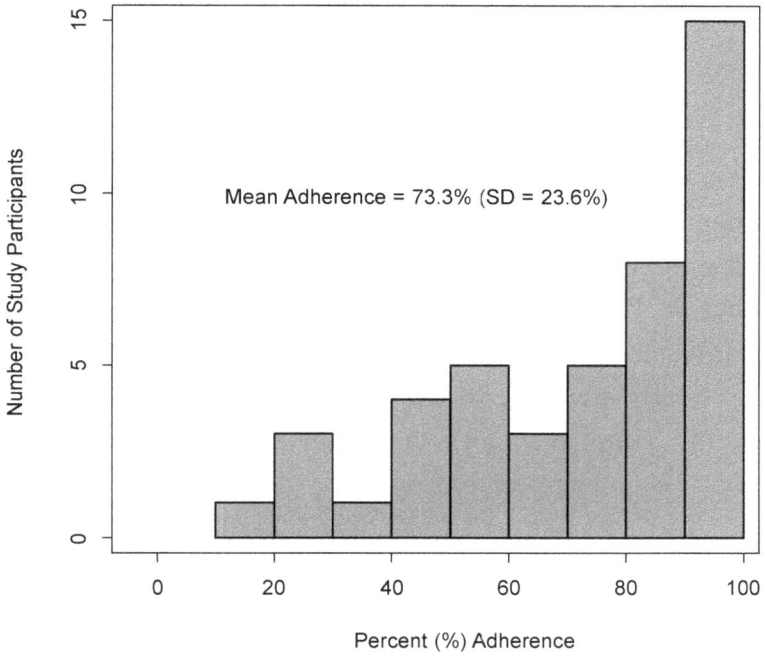

Mean Adherence = 73.3% (SD = 23.6%)

Number of Study Participants

Percent (%) Adherence

61

Figure 7. Correlations Between Individual DASS Subscales with BDI-II, BAI, and PSS-10 from Week 0 to 12 (N=47)

Scatter plots of change in DASS depression score versus change in BDI-II (A), change in DASS anxiety score versus change in BAI (B), change in DASS stress score versus change in PSS-10 (C) show highly statistically significant Spearman's rank correlation coefficients (ρ).

A positive change in score represents a decrease from baseline (improvement); a negative change in score represents an increase from baseline (decline).

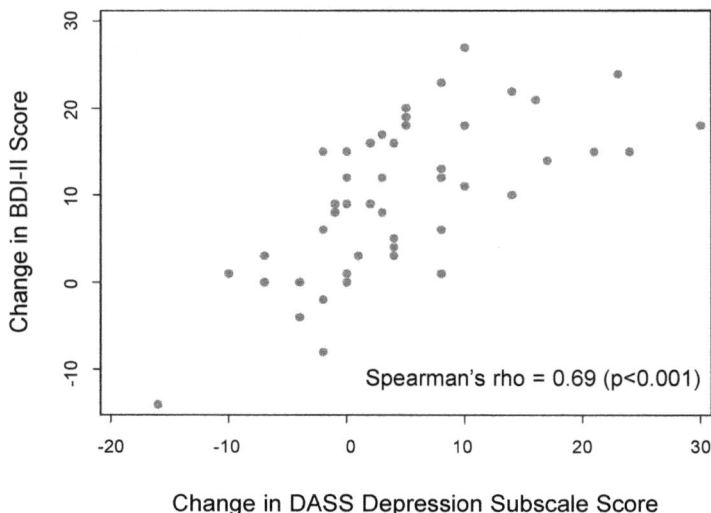

Spearman's rho = 0.69 (p<0.001)

Change in DASS Depression Subscale Score

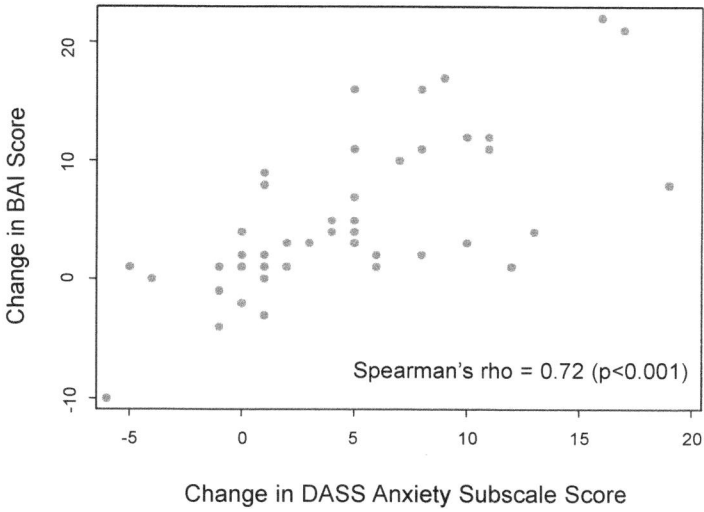

Spearman's rho = 0.72 (p<0.001)

Change in BAI Score

Change in DASS Anxiety Subscale Score

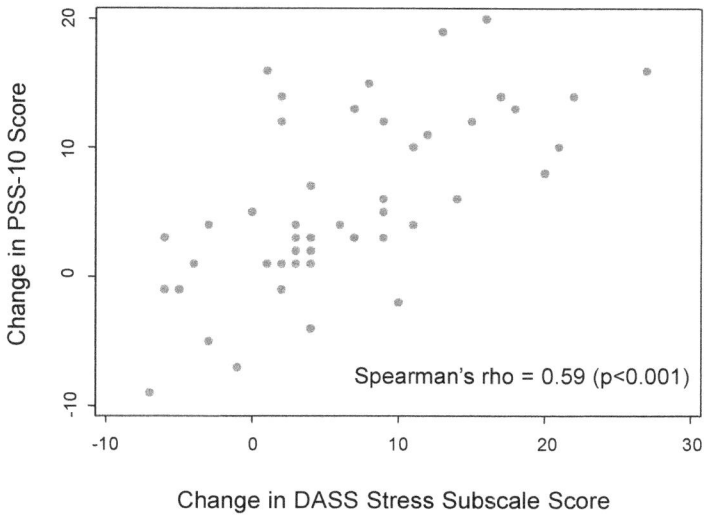

Spearman's rho = 0.59 (p<0.001)

Change in PSS-10 Score

Change in DASS Stress Subscale Score

REFERENCES

1. Guze SB (1992) *Why Psychiatry is a Branch of Medicine* New York, NY: Oxford University Press. 147p.

2. Lyness JM (1997) *Psychiatric Pearls.* Philadelphia, PA: F.A. Davis. 328p.

3. Storrow HA (1969) *Outline of Clinical Psychiatry.* New York, NY: Appleton-Century-Crofts. 535p.

4. Marneros A (2008) Psychiatry's 200th birthday. *Br J Psychiatry 193: 1-3.*

5. Kessler RC, Chiu WT, Demler O, Merikangas KR, Walters EE (2005) Prevalence, severity, and comorbidity of 12-month DSM-IV disorders in the National Comorbidity Survey Replication. *Arch Gen Psychiatry* 62: 617-627.

6. Collins MM, Corcoran P, Perry IJ (2009) Anxiety and depression symptoms in patients with diabetes. *Diabet Med* 26: 153-161.

7. Musselman DL, Betan E, Larsen H, Phillips LS (2003) Relationship of depression to diabetes types 1 and 2: epidemiology, biology, and treatment. *Biol Psychiatry* 54: 317-329.

8. Musselman DL, Evans DL, Nemeroff CB (1998) The relationship of depression to cardiovascular disease: epidemiology, biology, and treatment. *Arch Gen Psychiatry* 55: 580-592.

9. Shen BJ, Avivi YE, Todaro JF, Spiro AI, Laurenceau JP, et al. (2008) Anxiety characteristics independently and prospectively predict myocardial infarction in men: the unique contribution of anxiety among psychologic factors. *J Am Coll Cardiol* 51: 113-119.

10. Arnow BA, Blasey CM, Lee J, Fireman B, Hunkeler EM, et al. (2009) Relationships among depression, chronic pain, chronic disabling pain, and medical costs. *Psychiatr Serv* 60: 344-350.

11. Arnow BA, Hunkeler EM, Blasey CM, Lee J, Constantino MJ, et al. (2006) Comorbid depression, chronic pain, and disability in primary care. *Psychosom Med* 68: 262-268.

12. McWilliams LA, Cox BJ, Enns MW (2003) Mood and anxiety disorders associated with chronic pain: an examination in a nationally representative sample. *Pain* 106: 127-133.

13. Massie MJ (2004) Prevalence of depression in patients with cancer. *J Natl Cancer Inst Monogr*: 57-71.

14. Mitchell AJ, Chan M, Bhatti H, Halton M, Grassi L, et al. (2011) Prevalence of depression, anxiety, and adjustment disorder in oncological, haematological, and palliative-care settings: a meta-analysis of 94 interview-based studies. *Lancet Oncol* 12: 160-174.

15. Colibazzi T, Hsu TT, Gilmer WS (2006) Human immunodeficiency virus and depression in primary care: a clinical review. *Prim Care Companion J Clin Psychiatry* 8: 201-211.

16. Gunn JM, Ayton DR, Densley K, Pallant JF, Chondros P, et al. (2010) The association between chronic illness, multimorbidity and depressive symptoms in an Australian primary care cohort. *Soc Psychiatry Psychiatr Epidemiol*: 1-10.

17. Moussavi S, Chatterji S, Verdes E, Tandon A, Patel V, et al. (2007) Depression, chronic diseases, and decrements in health: results from the World Health Surveys. *Lancet* 370: 851-858.

18. Ciechanowski PS, Katon WJ, Russo JE (2000) Depression and diabetes: impact of depressive symptoms on adherence, function, and costs. *Arch Intern Med* 160: 3278-3285.

19. Gehi A, Haas D, Pipkin S, Whooley MA (2005) Depression and medication adherence in outpatients with coronary heart disease: findings from the Heart and Soul Study. *Arch Intern Med* 165: 2508-2513.

20. Whooley MA, de Jonge P, Vittinghoff E, Otte C, Moos R, et al. (2008) Depressive symptoms, health behaviors, and risk of cardiovascular events in patients with coronary heart disease. *JAMA* 300: 2379-2388.

21. Faris R, Purcell H, Henein MY, Coats AJ (2002) Clinical depression is common and significantly associated with reduced survival in patients with non-ischaemic heart failure. *Eur J Heart Fail* 4: 541-551.

22. Song EK, Lennie TA, Moser DK (2009) Depressive symptoms increase risk of rehospitalisation in heart failure patients with preserved systolic function. *J Clin Nurs* 18: 1871-1877.

23. Oxlad M, Stubberfield J, Stuklis R, Edwards J, Wade TD (2006) Psychological risk factors for increased post-operative length of hospital stay following coronary artery bypass graft surgery. *J Behav Med* 29: 179-190.

24. Mayou R (1991) Medically unexplained physical symptoms. *BMJ* 303: 534-535.

25. Brosschot JF, Gerin W, Thayer JF (2006) The perseverative cognition hypothesis: a review of worry, prolonged stress-related physiological activation, and health. *J Psychosom Res* 60: 113-124.

26. Verkuil B, Brosschot JF, Meerman EE, Thayer JF (2010) Effects of momentary assessed stressful events and worry episodes on somatic health complaints. *Psychol Health*: 1-18.

27. Jellesma FC, Verkuil B, Brosschot JF (2009) Postponing worrisome thoughts in children: the effects of a postponement intervention on perseverative thoughts, emotions and somatic complaints. *Soc Sci Med* 69: 278-284.

28. Tylee A, Gandhi P (2005) The importance of somatic symptoms in depression in primary care. *Prim Care Companion J Clin Psychiatry* 7: 167-176.

29. Cohen S, Janicki-Deverts D, Miller GE (2007) Psychological stress and disease. *JAMA* 298: 1685-1687.

30. Bereza BG, Machado M, Einarson TR (2009) Systematic review and quality assessment of economic evaluations and quality-of-life studies related to generalized anxiety disorder. *Clin Ther* 31: 1279-1308.

31. Burg M (1992) Stress, behavior, and heart disease. In: Zaret BL, Moser M, Cohen LS, editors. *Yale University School of Medicine Heart Book*. New York, NY: William Morrow and Co. pp. 95-104.

32. Saravay SM, Lavin M (1994) Psychiatric comorbidity and length of stay in the general hospital. A critical review of outcome studies. *Psychosomatics* 35: 233-252.

33. Sullivan M, Simon G, Spertus J, Russo J (2002) Depression-related costs in heart failure care. *Arch Intern Med* 162: 1860-1866.

34. Welch CA, Czerwinski D, Ghimire B, Bertsimas D (2009) Depression and costs of health care. *Psychosomatics* 50: 392-401.

35. McLaughlin KA, Nolen-Hoeksema S (2011) Rumination as a transdiagnostic factor in depression and anxiety. *Behav Res Ther* 49: 186-193.

36. Zoccola PM, Dickerson SS, Zaldivar FP (2008) Rumination and cortisol responses to laboratory stressors. *Psychosom Med* 70: 661-667.

37. Hecht D (2010) Depression and the hyperactive right-hemisphere. *Neurosci Res* 68: 77-87.

38. Hong RY (2007) Worry and rumination: differential associations with anxious and depressive symptoms and coping behavior. *Behav Res Ther* 45: 277-290.

39. Lyubomirsky S, Nolen-Hoeksema S (1995) Effects of self-focused rumination on negative thinking and interpersonal problem solving. *J Pers Soc Psychol* 69: 176-190.

40. Nolen-Hoeksema S (1991) Responses to depression and their effects on the duration of depressive episodes. *J Abnorm Psychol* 100: 569-582.

41. RW. Rathbun, personal communication (2005). Oceanside, CA.

42. Ward A, Lyubomirsky S, Sousa L, Nolen-Hoeksema S (2003) Can't quite commit: rumination and uncertainty. *Pers Soc Psychol Bull* 29: 96-107.

43. Zoccola PM, Dickerson SS, Lam S (2009) Rumination predicts longer sleep onset latency after an acute psychosocial stressor. *Psychosom Med* 71: 771-775.

44. Kiecolt-Glaser JK, McGuire L, Robles TF, Glaser R (2002) Emotions, morbidity, and mortality: new perspectives from psychoneuroimmunology. *Annu Rev Psychol* 53: 83-107.

45. Kubzansky LD, Kawachi I (2000) Going to the heart of the matter: do negative emotions cause coronary heart disease? *J Psychosom Res* 48: 323-337.

46. Larzelere MM, Jones GN (2008) Stress and health. *Prim Care Clin Office Pract* 35: 839-856.

47. Sirois BC, Burg MM (2003) Negative emotion and coronary heart disease. A review. *Behav Modif* 27: 83-102.

48. Bennett EJ, Tennant CC, Piesse C, Badcock CA, Kellow JE (1998) Level of chronic life stress predicts clinical outcome in irritable bowel syndrome. *Gut* 43: 256-261.

49. Massey EK, Garnefski N, Gebhardt WA, van der Leeden R (2011) A daily diary study on the independent and interactive effects of headache and self-regulatory factors on daily affect among adolescents. *Br J Health Psychol* 16: 288-299.

50. Gerin W, Davidson KW, Christenfeld NJ, Goyal T, Schwartz JE (2006) The role of angry rumination and distraction in blood pressure recovery from emotional arousal. *Psychosom Med* 68: 64-72.

51. Harburg E, Julius M, Kaciroti N, Gleiberman L, Schork MA (2003) Expressive/suppressive anger-coping responses, gender, and types of mortality: a 17-year follow-up (Tecumseh, Michigan, 1971-1988). *Psychosom Med* 65: 588-597.

52. Anisman H, Merali Z (2002) Cytokines, stress, and depressive illness. *Brain Behav Immun* 16: 513-524.

53. Habib KE, Gold PW, Chrousos GP (2001) Neuroendocrinology of stress. Endocrinol Metab *Clin North Am* 30: 695-728.

54. Holsboer F (1995) Neuroendocrinology of mood disorders. In: Bloom FE, Kupfer DJ, editors. *Psychopharmacology: The Fourth Generation of Progress.* New York, NY: Raven Press. pp. 970-982.

55. McEwen BS, Gianaros PJ (2011) Stress- and allostasis-induced brain plasticity. *Annu Rev Med* 62: 431-445.

56. Tsigos C, Chrousos GP (2002) Hypothalamic-pituitary-adrenal axis, neuroendocrine factors and stress. *J Psychosom Res* 53: 865-871.

57. Covington HE, 3rd, Maze I, LaPlant QC, Vialou VF, Ohnishi YN, et al. (2009) Antidepressant actions of histone deacetylase inhibitors. *J Neurosci* 29: 11451-11460.

58. Renthal W, Maze I, Krishnan V, Covington HE, 3rd, Xiao G, et al. (2007) Histone deacetylase 5 epigenetically controls behavioral adaptations to chronic emotional stimuli. *Neuron* 56: 517-529.

59. Tsankova N, Renthal W, Kumar A, Nestler EJ (2007) Epigenetic regulation in psychiatric disorders. *Nat Rev Neurosci* 8: 355-367.

60. Xie P, Kranzler HR, Poling J, Stein MB, Anton RF, et al. (2010) Interaction of FKBP5 with childhood adversity on risk for post-traumatic stress disorder. *Neuropsychopharmacology* 35: 1684-1692.

61. Lupien SJ, Maheu F, Tu M, Fiocco A, Schramek TE (2007) The effects of stress and stress hormones on human cognition: implications for the field of brain and cognition. *Brain Cogn* 65: 209-237.

62. McEwen BS (2007) Physiology and neurobiology of stress and adaptation: central role of the brain. *Physiol Rev* 87: 873-904.

63. Bjorntorp P (2001) Do stress reactions cause abdominal obesity and comorbidities? *Obes Rev* 2: 73-86.

64. Rathbun RW (2007) *The Kelee: An Understanding of the Psychology of Spirituality*. Oceanside, CA: Quiescence Publishing. 369p.

65. Rathbun RW (2008) *The Kelee Meditation Practice: The Basic Principles of the Kelee*. Oceanside, CA: Quiescence Publishing. 56p.

66. Rathbun RW (2010) *Troubleshooting the Mind: Understanding the Basic Principles of the Kelee*. Oceanside, CA: Quiescence Publishing. 224p.

67. Rathbun RW. Kelee Foundation Web site (2012). www.thekelee.org. Accessed: March 12, 2012.

68. Rathbun RW (2007) *The Way is Within: A Spiritual Journey*. Oceanside, CA: Quiescence Publishing. 276p.

69. Rathbun RW (2011) *The Silent Miracle: Awakening Your True Spiritual Nature*. Oceanside, CA: Quiescence Publishing. 300p.

70. Rathbun RW (2011) *The Mind and Self-Reflection: A New Way to Read with Your Mind.* Oceanside, CA: Quiescence Publishing. 278p.

71. Lovibond SH, Lovibond PF (1995) *Manual for the Depression Anxiety and Stress Scales.* Sydney, Australia: Psychology Foundation. 42p.

72. Beck AT, Steer RA, Brown GK (1996) *Manual for the Beck Depression Inventory-II.* San Antonio, TX: Psychological Corporation. 38p.

73. Beck AT, Steer RA (1990) *Manual for the Beck Anxiety Inventory.* San Antonio, TX: Psychological Corporation. 23p.

74. Cohen S, Williamson G (1988) The social psychology of health: Claremont Symposium on applied social psychology. In: Spacapan S, Oskamp S, editors. *Perceived Stress in a Probability Sample of the United States.* Newbury Park, CA: Sage. pp. 31-67.

75. Derogatis LR (1994) SCL-90-R: *Administration, Scoring and Procedures Manual.* Minneapolis, MN: NCS Pearson. 119p.

76. Ware JE, Snow KK, Konsinki M, Gandek B (1993) *SF-36 Health Survey Manual and Interpretation Guide.* Boston, MA: The Health Institute.

77. Ware JE, Kosinski M (2002) SF-36 *Physical and Mental Health Summary Scales: A Manual for Users of Version 1, Second Edition*. Lincoln, Rhode Island: QualityMetric Incorporated. 237p.

78. World Health Organization (1946) Preamble to the constitution of the World Health Organization. *Constitution of the World Health Organization*. Geneva, Switzerland: World Health Organization. pp.2.

79. Roy-Byrne PP, Davidson KW, Kessler RC, Asmundson GJ, Goodwin RD, et al. (2008) Anxiety disorders and comorbid medical illness. *Gen Hosp Psychiatry* 30: 208-225.

80. Means-Christensen AJ, Roy-Byrne PP, Sherbourne CD, Craske MG, Stein MB (2008) Relationships among pain, anxiety, and depression in primary care. *Depress Anxiety* 25: 593-600.

81. Sareen J, Cox BJ, Clara I, Asmundson GJ (2005) The relationship between anxiety disorders and physical disorders in the U.S. National Comorbidity Survey. *Depress Anxiety* 21: 193-202.

82. Levenstein S (2000) The very model of a modern etiology: a biopsychosocial view of peptic ulcer. *Psychosom Med* 62: 176-185.

ACKNOWLEDGMENTS

The authors would like to thank several individuals for their contributions to the completion of this study. We would like to acknowledge Moira Mar-Tang for the coordination of the entire study (including screening of study participants, coordination of Kelee classes, administering the questionnaires, and acquiring the data). We would also like to thank Amy Sitapati, MD for her assistance with study design and data analysis.

In addition, the authors would like to acknowledge Frank A. Silva for his assistance in teaching all of the Kelee classes, Lavana Rathbun, Nikki Walsh for her assistance with the figures, Anita C. Smith and Tari L. Gilbert for their assistance with administering the semi-structured interviews, Joanna M. Phillips, Kenneth E. Bonus, and Freeman L. Sands Jr., for their assistance in reviewing the final manuscript.

Funding Support

This Kelee meditation study was funded by the UCSD Academic Senate Grant (Grant#: RK084H-LEE, RL155M-LEE, http://senate.ucsd.edu/cor/calls/HSresearch.htm). These two grants were utilized to cover transcription costs for semi-structured qualitative interviews, of which this data will be presented in a separate, future manuscript. Research support in the form of data analysis (including power calculations) was provided by UCSD Center for AIDS Research (Grant#: AI36214, http://cfar.ucsd.edu/).

There are no commercial sponsors nor was this study funded by the Kelee Foundation or Being Alive San Diego. The funders had no role in study design, data collection and analysis, decision to publish, or preparation of the manuscript.

Competing Interests

The Principal Investigator, Daniel Lee (DL), and his study team have donated their time and efforts toward determining the usefulness of Kelee meditation. There was no compensation or payment provided to the study participants or investigators for completion of this study. All study participants, regardless of their primary care provider, entered the study on their own accord. There was no compensation provided to either the Kelee Foundation (KF) or Being Alive San Diego (BASD) for the use of its facility for the meditation classes. Both entities are non-profit 501(c)(3) organizations.

DL does not have any financial interest or investment in the KF, nor is he a paid or in-kind consultant for this organization. However, he has made financial donations to the KF on his own behalf. His only affiliation with KF is as a student of Kelee meditation. He has been paying for private sessions for spiritual guidance with Mr. Ron W. Rathbun (Founder of the KF) for over 7 years.

DL has voluntarily written a testimonial for the KF website (www.thekelee.org) and 2 forewords for books written by Mr. Ron W. Rathbun. As a physician, DL has offered Kelee meditation as another tool to help patients with stress, anxiety, and depression. He has purchased Kelee meditation books and given them freely to patients interested in meditation. DL participated in recruiting patients for this study, but he did not provide special incentives for his own patients or any other patients to enter the study.

Furthermore, he has also donated dozens of books to BASD (site of the meditation classes). DL currently serves as the Board President for BASD for several years and has been on the Board of Directors for BASD for over 12 years. As a board member of BASD, there is a financial relationship as the board is required to provide fiduciary oversight of the organization. However, DL is not a paid employee of BASD but volunteers his time and effort. He has made numerous financial donations to BASD on his own accord. Of note, DL donated the books used in this study.

AFTERWORD

As someone who has continued to practice Kelee meditation for over 7½ years, I am amazed at the continual improvement in the quality of my own personal life in regards to stress, anxiety, and depression. It was these personal improvements that inspired me to study Kelee meditation in patients who were struggling with these same issues.

The quantitative results of the study speak for themselves. Highly statistically significant improvements in stress, anxiety, and depression were seen across multiple standardized questionnaires in just 12 short weeks. But what is even more amazing than this data is how patients qualitatively felt on a mental level after just 12 weeks. The results of the qualitative semi-structured interviews and longitudinal data out to 52 weeks will be presented separately in the near future.

Since completion of this study, I have been asked why the investigators chose not to use a control arm. Well, if you think about it, Kelee meditation teaches you to develop stillness (the absence of distraction from thoughts and the 5 physical senses), which is actually the purest form of a non-intervention. What is a control arm to a non-intervention? There really is none. Keep in mind that this issue regarding the lack of a control arm is particular to this study only.[41]

Kelee meditation is unique in this manner, as the goal is to not to do anything, just to be. Thus, creating an intervention, such as a sham meditation is useless as a comparison. The closest thing to a comparison arm is really everyone who is not doing Kelee meditation. Thus, any improvements seen with doing Kelee meditation is really due to Kelee meditation.[41]

The real advantage of Kelee meditation compared to other interventions for improving mental health is that we are not introducing a medication nor are we trying to change someone's thoughts in order to change how someone feels. Participants are asked only to still their mind and to practice essentially "doing" nothing, which is just "being". As a result, there are no side effects from introduction of a chemical in the body, nor necessarily the creation of mental resistance by trying to introduce new thoughts. This is what is impressive about our results.[41]

On a personal note, I have continued to find more benefits of developing a still mind from Kelee meditation, which has translated to everything I do, including my work with patients. As an active practicing physician working with patients, I am keenly aware of the amount of stress related to patient care and working in healthcare. I can honestly say that I am much more focused, efficient, and less affected these days by my work as a physician despite the push in healthcare to be more productive. I feel that I am able to use my developed self-awareness and perception to better understand what is going on with my patients on a mental and physical level. Kelee meditation has taught me how to care about myself through the self-understanding of what has caused me to take in negative thoughts and emotion that detract from my quality of life.

More recently, I have begun to understand that it is through caring for ourselves first that allows us to extend this feeling of caring to others. The ability to care and provide help to others is a beautiful quality to have as a medical provider, but it is achieved most effectively if we are in a detached space (unaffected by negative emotion). Kelee meditation teaches how to stop looping and to dissolve our compartments, so we can learn how to live in a space of detachment. This, in turn, allows us to care for others, but not become affected adversely in the process.[41]

How often are you affected by the care that you provide to your patients? What is learning to get to the state of detachment worth to you? With this in mind, I have recently embarked on another study looking at using Kelee meditation for reducing job burnout in nurses, which is a huge issue in healthcare. We are also planning on introducing Kelee meditation in medical school curricula to also help students and residents develop another tool to work with patients in the health care setting. Stay tuned for future developments.

I would seriously encourage anyone and everyone to give Kelee meditation a try and to experience what Kelee meditation can do for you. All it takes is 5-10 minutes twice daily to learn how to still your mind. You have nothing to lose by trying and everything to gain (and more…)!

Daniel Lee, MD
Clinical Professor of Medicine
UCSD School of Medicine
UCSD Medical Center–Owen Clinic
May 2013